I0791672

BLOOM AT 85

A Guide to Happy Healthy Longevity

Alan Bloom

BALBOA.PRESS

A DIVISION OF HAY HOUSE

Balboa Press books may be ordered through booksellers or by contacting:

Balboa Press
A Division of Hay House
1663 Liberty Drive
Bloomington, IN 47403
www.balboapress.co.uk
UK TFN: 0800 0148647 (Toll Free inside the UK)
UK Local: 02036 956325 (+44 20 3695 6325 from outside the UK)

Print information available on the last page.

ISBN: 978-1-9822-8253-0 (sc)
ISBN: 978-1-9822-8254-7 (e)

Balboa Press rev. date: 01/27/2021

(An 85 year old gives you perspective to happy healthy longevity)

How did I get to 85 years old and without being on any prescribed medications?

Find out the secrets that helped me reach 85 years old without taking any long term drugs, and keeping in great physical and mental shape.

There's a whole new life waiting for you, if you want it.

<u>THIS IS A SELF HELP BOOK</u>

ACKNOWLEDGMENT

My son Richard Bloom who helped me with all the IT, and was my camera man.

My daughter Alison Bloom who proof read the book.

Thank you.

PREFACE

Sadly in 2019 Alan's wife Josephine passed away, and he decided to move into a retirement community where he could live on his own, but still be in contact with people in a communal lounge when he wanted some company. He was disturbed to see how many of the residents were disabled, and to find that some of them hardly ever left their apartments to socialise. They seemed to be just living a lonely life of survival and 'waiting for God.'

This book has been written for all the people who want to keep healthy and don't want to lose their motivation for life when they enter retirement, and possibly miss out in a new and wonderful stage in it.

MOVING INTO RETIREMENT

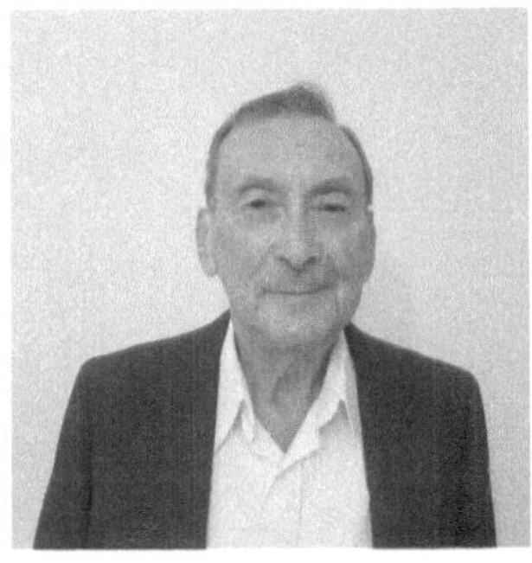 STAYING active, being happy, and keeping healthy is the key to enjoying old age. Traditionally, people wanted a retirement where doing almost nothing was the goal, enjoying a leisurely slide into death. They felt they had earned this from years of hard work.

I feel that retirement is a unique opportunity to experience a new life. I wanted this book to give you the tools to enable you to achieve a retirement as good or better than my own.

WORKING FOR YOURSELF

When people retire they think they are on holiday all the time. What do you do on holiday? You eat to excess, drink to excess, you lounge around and only do the things you want to do.

This holiday mentality is insidious. Why? Because it can and will become the norm and you find yourself five years later in hospital suffering from ill health. Yes, it's good to have a holiday, maybe a month or two, but not a permanent one, because it is not going to feel like a holiday anymore.

I believe that you can ONLY truly enjoy yourself when you feel well. However, this means that people must return from their holiday and go back to 'work'. Now you have a new full-time job. What is your new job? It is looking after your own health, but it is not working for anybody else, it is working for yourself.

What you eat, what you drink, and above all the exercise you do to keep strong and flexible should now be your priority. You should create a routine to live by.

People are living longer for many reasons. There are new medical breakthroughs happening all the time. The quality of life is improving. Living space is getting better. We have more knowledge about foods and what keeps us healthy. We know about vitamin supplements and nutrition. But if we want to live to a 'ripe old age' and be active right up to the end, we have to do more.

I have found that the next most important thing to diet is NOT stimulating the brain with puzzles and games, but building up the muscles of the body.

Without a healthy body everything else will become useless. Exercise not only keeps you flexible it helps circulate the vascular (blood) system which in turn helps everything else, the heart, the lungs, the brain, and the organs etc. (see Weight Training).

Slowing down and relaxing after retirement is expected, but the best part is whatever you want to do, you can do in your own time.

I don't sit around for any length of time, your body doesn't like to sit around for too long, I always get up and walk around within an hour or less, and I keep at least half-an-hour a day for walking out and stretching my legs.

You should create a fresh routine to live by, and stick to it. Allowing the subconscious mind to do things automatically, and freeing up the conscious mind to think of interesting things to do. Get up at a reasonable time in the morning and keep to the same time each day. You can still eat the same type of food but maybe reduce the quantity, because you are not burning it off so much. Keep in mind older people should eat more protein and less carbohydrate than younger people. Eating vegetables and fruit is also very beneficial.

Try and take full responsibility for your own health, don't leave it to the doctor. This could be your new job. It will give you something to aim for. It will give you the encouragement to look forward to a happy new life, and give you a reason to get up in the mornings. To know the joy of physical well being, and to do things you've always wanted to do but never had the time. The chance to be active and enjoy life right up until it's your time to go, instead of wasting away slowly in a care home, and suffering the indignities of people feeding you, dressing you, washing you, etc., until you just fade away. It doesn't have to be that way, and it might take a lot longer than you anticipated.

INTRODUCTION

HEALTH is the key to enjoying old age. How do we do this? You may be retired from your last job, or about to be. People look at their retirement as a time to take it easy, to stop doing almost everything except maybe a bit of gardening, or not even that, and that is the worst thing they can do. The body does not work like that. If you don't use it, you lose it, and pretty soon everything starts falling apart. But if you look upon your retirement as a new job or a new hobby, and consider your health as the most important part of it, it will give you a reason for you to get up in the morning, a reason to exercise in order to be strong and flexible. You should create a routine to live by, so that you do it without thinking. Human beings work better when they are in a routine. For example, if you normally eat breakfast before you go to work then you should continue to do so. Some people just have tea or coffee and a slice of toast. That's alright, if that's what you've wanted to do, whatever you decide, stick with it. The only difference, as I've said before, is that older people should have more protein and less carbohydrates than younger people.

Perhaps you would like to travel. Of course you've got to be able to afford it, but you've got to be fit enough to do it as well. Being fit will give you encouragement to look forward to holidays, going to live entertainment, enjoying physical well-being, and a reason to want to live. It is important to adopt a healthy lifestyle. Universities encourage sport. Why? Because it not only keeps the body fit, but actually aids brain function. Many older people think that as long as you exercise the brain you will live longer. They read books, do puzzles and crosswords, and play board games, and think that is sufficient, it isn`t. In my opinion, physical health is the most important factor.

Most people believe that diet is the way to a longer active life, well it is partially correct, but although a sensible diet is important, exercise is even more critical. ***If you don't use it you you lose it.*** The problem is that as you get older you naturally lose cells, and by the time you are 80 you lose something like 50% of your muscle. Just doing exercise won`t bring it back, but there is a way of reversing it, or at least slowing down the degeneration, which has not been taken seriously enough and hardly mentioned.

The body loves resistance as well as exercise. I have discovered the older we get, the more exercise we require. Have you noticed how stiff you are when you get out of bed in the morning, because the body does not like staying still for a long time? It's like a car doesnt like being stationary for a long period, the fluids solidify. You should never sit still for more than an hour, even if it's only to get up to make a cup of tea. The body loves walking briskly (not running), any activity is good. Gardening is a very popular way to keep active, but of course not everyone likes it, or even has a garden. Fishing is not so beneficial, as you stay inactive for long periods. Cycling has become more popular recently, but although it is a nice way to keep fit, it can be quite dangerous, especially for the elderly. You can go to the gym, but that has its limitations, like the amount of time you can spend doing it, travelling to get there, limited opening times, plus the expense.

When I was sixty-eight, my son decided to move to Spain with his wife and little boy. He liked to keep himself fit, and he left us with a set of free hand weights which were too cumbersome to take with him. And so I began to use them, they were pairs of 1 kilo, 2 kilo and 3 kilo weights. I found a book on weight training (not weight lifting), and started with the smallest ones. In a relatively short time, I started to feel the benefits. I felt more flexible, my arms and lungs felt stronger, I was standing more upright, and had an overall feeling of well being. I did it about twice a week. At the same time I did quite a bit of walking, and when it rained, I ran up and down the internal stairway of the building that I lived in for exercise. I have been doing regular exercise ever since, and walking one to two miles most days.

I AM 85 years old, I am not on any medications of any sort. However, I did have total kidney failure 11 years ago. I was on the dialysis machine for over a month, and no-one expected me to survive. I did survive, and what's more, after being on steroids for over four years, my kidneys are now in excellent shape. I put my recovery down to my general fitness, and help from my son who is a hypnotherapist. I have all my faculties, although I do need hearing aids and spectacles. I do exercise, and walk up to an hour every day, and more importantly, I do weight training. In case you think that it is genetics that has given me this healthy longevity, I can tell you that my mother had four brothers, and my father was one of three brothers. Only one of the men in my family got past the age of 75 - that was my mother's brother who was a keen sportsman and died at the age of 86.

When I retired at 65, we moved to a retirement block by the sea. It was there my wife met a lady who played green bowls, and she invited my wife to try it. Well my wife really enjoyed it. It was a bowls club with separate sections for men and women. She not only enjoyed playing the game, but also the social side, as most of the members were of a similar age to us. After a short time she persuaded me to join the men's section. We played three times a week for home games, and more if we played against other clubs. So it kept us pretty active. We were in a league of about nine clubs, and met up with many people. It was a good decision, and we've been playing bowls for almost twenty years.

HEALTHY EATING

When people talk about reaching an active 80+, they usually put it down to a sensible diet. It is the cornerstone to good health, but it has to be the one that is best for you, not because its what you like to eat, but what you think is the healthiest food for you. We are all different when it comes to food. Lots of us have allergies, and we have to find out what is right for us personally. I can give you some tips, but it is up to the reader to find the diet that works for them.

Beef, lamb and pork are not recommended as they contain substances that block up blood vessels. I mostly eat fish (three times a week). Oily fish such as salmon, sardines, herring, and mackerel are particularly good for you. I have chicken quite frequently too. I also eat some of the processed vegetarian foods such as Quorn, and Linda McCartney, (*There are lots of other products available*). It is recommended that the older you are, the more protein you should eat, like fish, cheese, eggs, poultry, and less carbohydrates like potatoes, bread, and pasta. Rice is a good substitute and it is a protein. I try to eat a reasonable amount of fruit, salad and veg most days. Eat your food slowly, and chew it well, at least 20 to 30 times. Many people don't chew their food long enough, which causes indegestion.You need to reduce the quantity of food you eat as well, because you're not burning as many calories.

I have cereal for breakfast, I use four different ones, and I like to mix them. For example, I have slices of banana and berries or grapes with the cereal. Occasionally I have porridge. It seems to work well for me, as my bowels are usually pretty good. Processed food such as bacon, sausages, and burgers I have only moderately. Fruit should be eaten at least half-an-hour before main meals and one hour afterwards to avoid mixing with other fluids in the stomach. Drink after a meal, not during, because it dilutes the acid in the stomach that breaks down the food during digestion. That old saying, 'Breakfast like a prince, lunch like a king, and supper like a pauper' is worth bearing in mind. Avoid eating large meals at night, because you are making your digestive system work hard while you are sleeping, and you are not giving your body the rest it needs.

Keep sugar and salt to a minimum, both of these are poisonous to the system. Too much sugar can cause diabetes type 2, weight gain, and cancer. There are two types of diabetes, type 1 is given to us by our inheritance from the family we are born into. Diabetes 2 we give to ourselves, and is a very serious condition. As we get older our organs become less efficient. The pancreas, which makes insulin to control the sugar in the body, and is part of the digestive system, becomes less efficient with age. It works if you don't overload it, but if you give it too much to do, (large amounts of food or sugar), it will eventually give up, and that is called diabetes 2. Too much salt can raise blood pressure which can put greater strain on the heart, and that can cause heart attacks, strokes, kidney disease, and damage to the brain. No table salt, but Celtic sea salt which contains ten minerals is actually recommended.

Keep alcohol down to a minimum - in spite of what people say to the contrary, it might be good for the soul, but it is not so good for the body. Just one beer or a glass of wine a day, perhaps. A small glass of whisky or brandy mixed with water, of an evening, can be therapeutic. Drinking small amounts of water throughout the day up to about 2 litres is really important, but not in the evening, as it will keep you up during the night.

PHYSICAL FITNESS

The next most important part of this new beginning is to build up physical strength. Without this nothing can be achieved, and you will slowly waste away. The body needs strength and flexibility. I have discovered the older we get, the more exercise we require. No-one ever told me that before. There are 600 muscles in the body. If you don't use them they will eventually seize up. Have you noticed how stiff you get in the morning when you've just got out of bed? This is because the body doesn't like keeping still for any length of time. At the risk of repeating myself, you must never sit for more than an hour without getting up and moving around, even if it's only to make a cup of tea.

EXERCISE

Have you noticed when cats wake up they have a bout of stretching? Well we should do the same. Before we do any of the proper exercises, stretch your arms out in front of you. Pick a point directly behind you. Bring your right arm up slowly from your side up to eye level. With your palm facing outwards, and keeping your eyes on that hand all of the time, slowly move your straight arm out to the side and swing out and around to the back to that fixed point, keeping your feet firmly facing forward so that you have to twist the rest of your body around to watch your hand go directly behind you to the fixed point. Do this several times alternating hands, and raising and pushing your hand further above your head each time. This exercises your arms, your neck, and your eyes all at the same time, and will help you to keep flexible. Then kick your legs out to the side alternately, like the Japanese Sumo wrestlers. This part of a warm up. Do this every day.

The body likes walking, cycling, swimming, and recent research has found that dancing is the best exercise of all, plus yoga type exercises. Running is not recommended for older people. It is not necessary to go to a gym for exercise. You can have everything you need in your own home, where you can do it more frequently, and at no cost. If you have stairs available or close by, use them in your exercise routine. They are very good for the legs, the heart, and the lungs. If you are worried about what exercises to do, there are many books on it, or you can look on YouTube where there are lots of exercise videos to be had, and you can select what suits you. Do not overexert yourself. Start off very slowly with very short workouts, and always give yourself several minutes for your heart to slow down between exercises. Start weight training once a week to give your muscles a chance to get used to it. You will probably ache the first few times. Wear warmish comfortable clothing like a track suit, to keep the muscles warm. Always try to maintain an even temperature. Never get too cold, or too hot. Having flexed and warmed up the muscles in your arms and legs with various exercises for about twenty minutes, we can now move on to the weights.

WEIGHT TRAINING

What I am about to explain may seem simplistic but I assure you it really does work, and I am living proof of it. The body thrives on resistance. The more it gets, the stronger it becomes. It doesn't matter what kind of resistance, it could be swimming, cycling, or even mountain climbing. However, I have found that the most convenient discipline for me is weight training. By moving your arms around holding these weights you can stimulate the heart, increase lung capacity, massage the internal organs, enlarge the muscles, send more oxygen to the brain through blood circulation, tighten up your stomach muscles, which help to support your back and help digestion, give you a feeling of general well being, increase testosterone, and regenerate your libido. And it can be done at home. It is much safer than the other ways, and is the most suitable for older people. What is needed is a combination of exercises and weight training, and the older you are the more frequent it has to be. This is because as we get older our joints freeze up quicker. It is not necessary to go to a gym to do weight training. I started going to one, and didn't like it. I prefer to do it on my own. I can do it when I want to, how I want to, as often as I wish, and at no cost, except for the initial purchase of the weights.

For a small outlay, you can buy a set of free hand weights, they are normally available from somewhere like Argos, Amazon, or Ebay. I started with a set of three pairs of plastic covered hand weights 1 kilo, 2kilos, and 4kilos. People usually start with 1 kilo and as you become stronger you move to the heavier ones, I am now using 4.5 kilo weights' which is not bad for an eighty-five year old! You don't have to strain too much, as soon as it becomes uncomfortable, you stop. It's more about repetition than lifting heavy weights. You can buy books on weight training, and there are many good videos on YouTube teaching you how to do exercises and use free weights.I have a yoga mat to lie on, when I do lifting while lying on my back. As I said earlier, I started with 1 kilo weights and gradually increased them over the years as I became stronger. I have also increased the number of workouts per week. At first it was once a week, then twice a week, then in my late seventies, it was three times a week, or every other day, and since I have reached eighty, it has been every day. The logic is that if you can make your muscles strong enough to move weights around, it's going to be much easier for your limbs to move around without them. I am now actually stronger than I was 20 years ago, and more flexible. Weight training not only strengthens the arms and legs, it also helps the internal organs such as the heart, the lungs, the stomach. And sends oxygen via the blood to the brain.

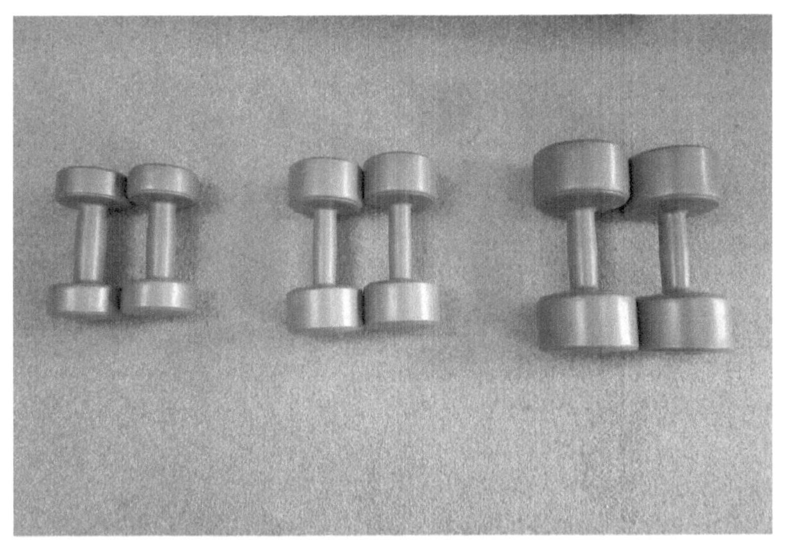

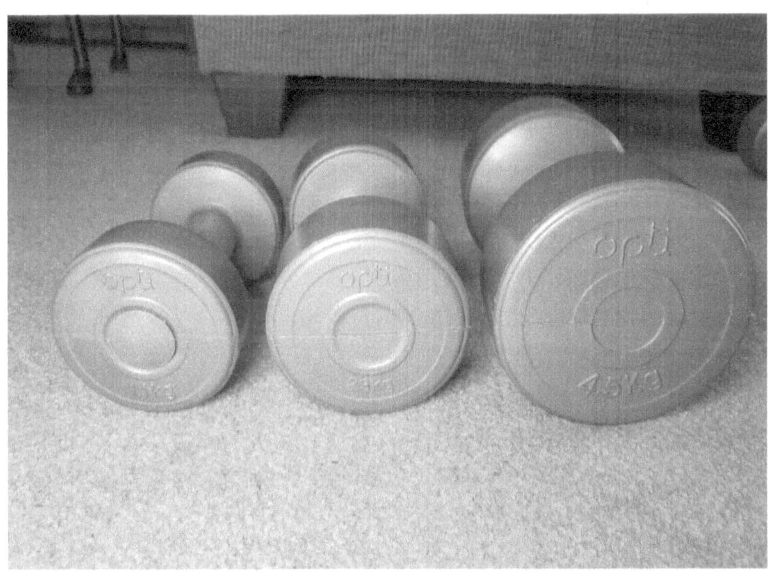

opb
opb
opb

WEIGHT TRAINING (WT)

WT Stimulates all the organs
WT Increases testosterone
WT Improves libido
WT Increases overall strength
WT Stimulates the blood circulation
WT Strengthens the heart
WT Strengthens the lungs
WT Protects from osteoporosis
WT Helps prevent arthritis
WT Improves flexibility
WT Helps bowel movement
WT Strengthens bones
WT Enlarges the muscles
WT Encourages healthy eating
WT Improves appearance
WT Stimulates the brain
WT Boosts confidence
WT Lowers cholesterol
WT Helps you sleep better
WT Wards off dementia
WT Gives you the 'feel young' factor

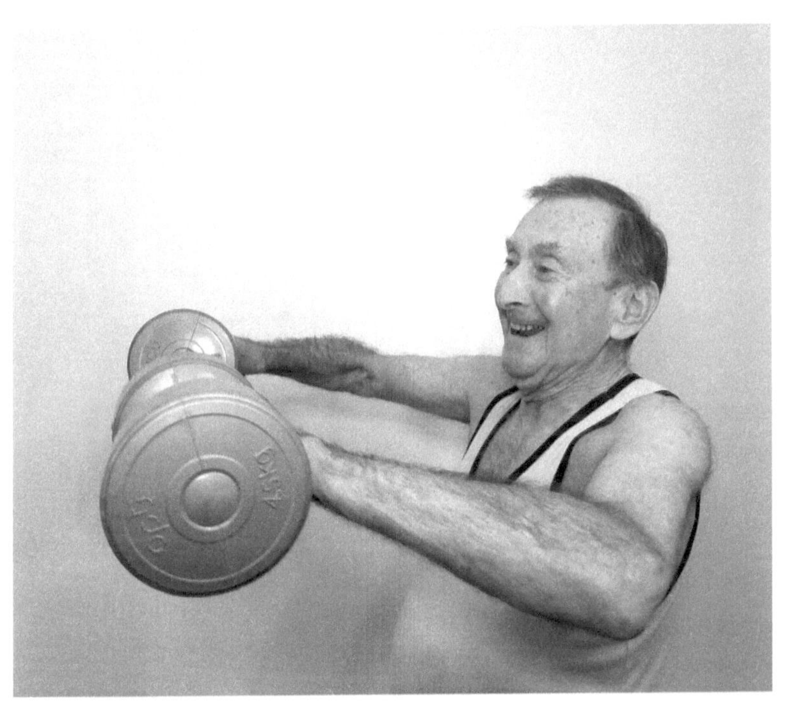

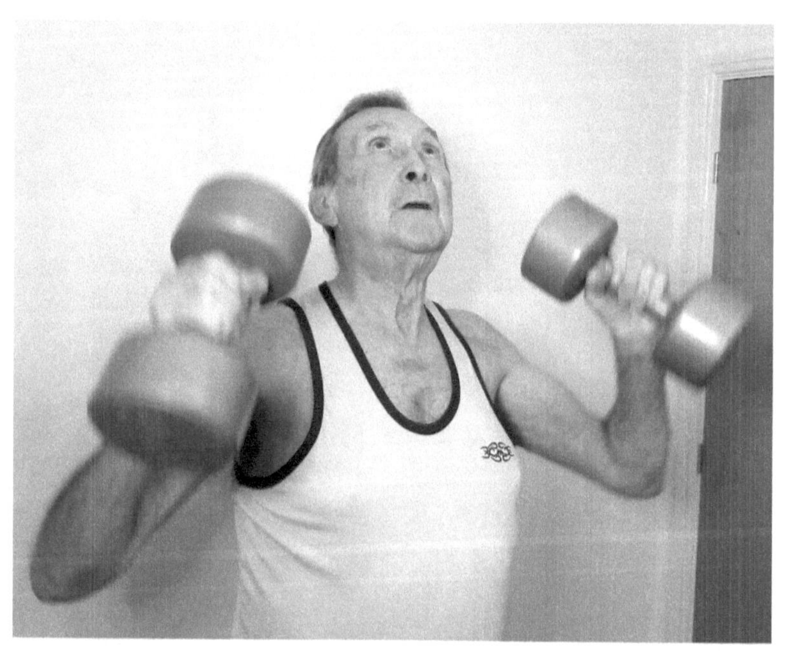

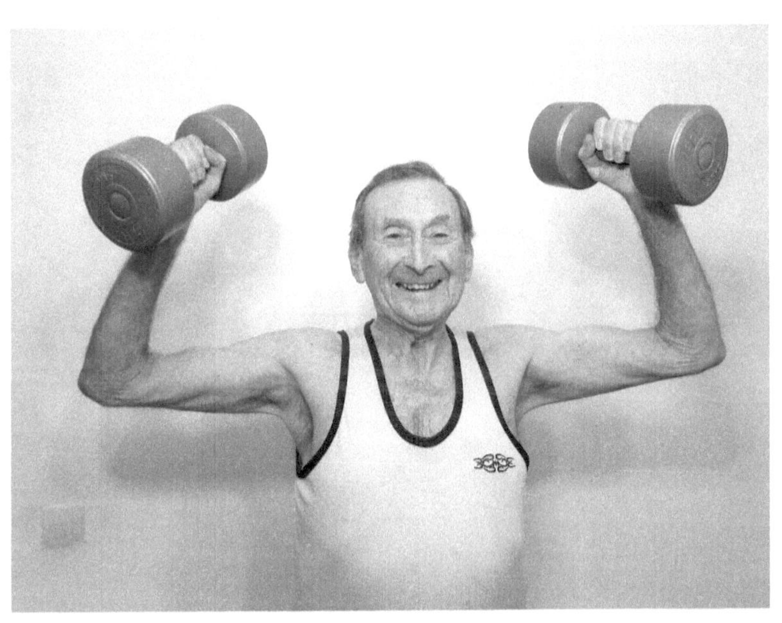

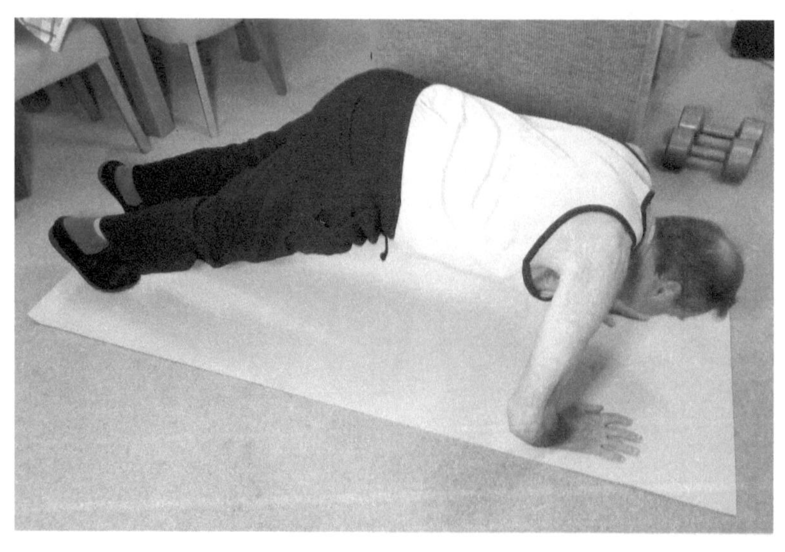

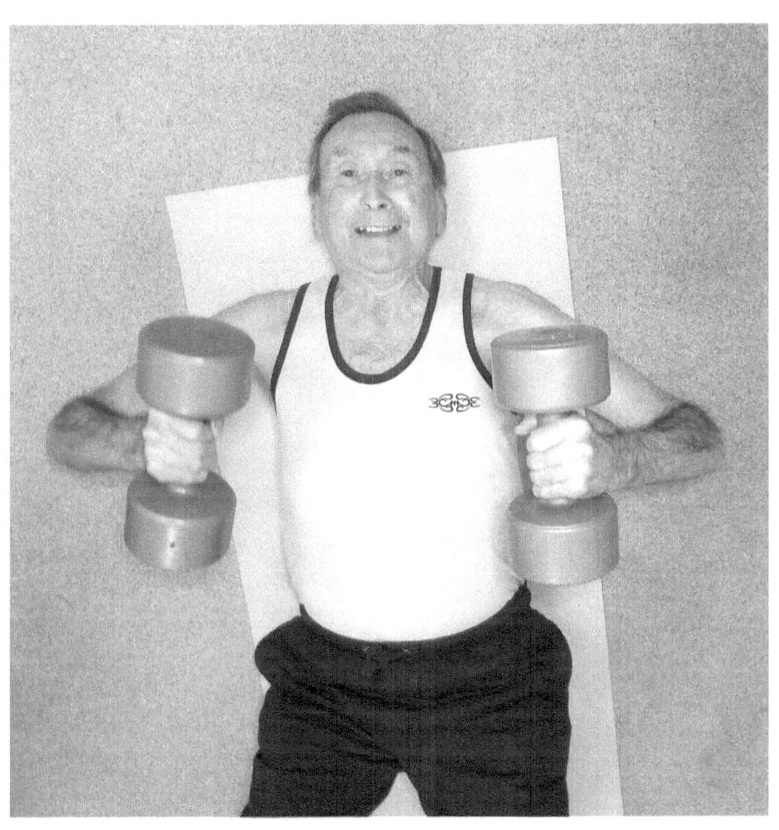

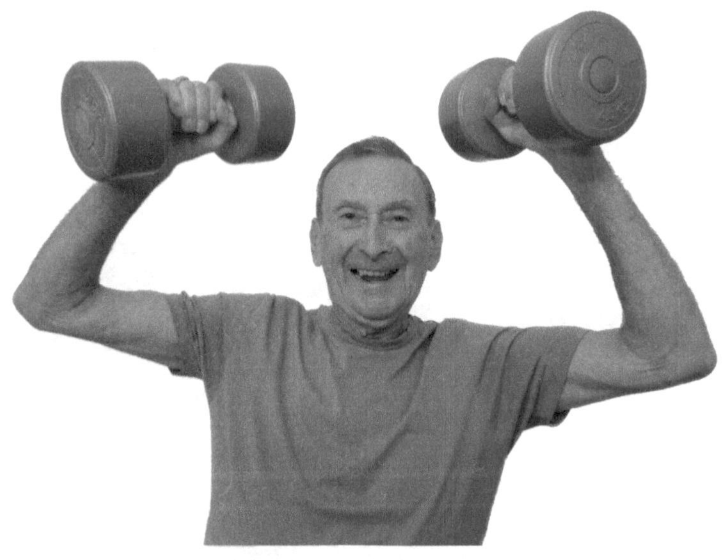

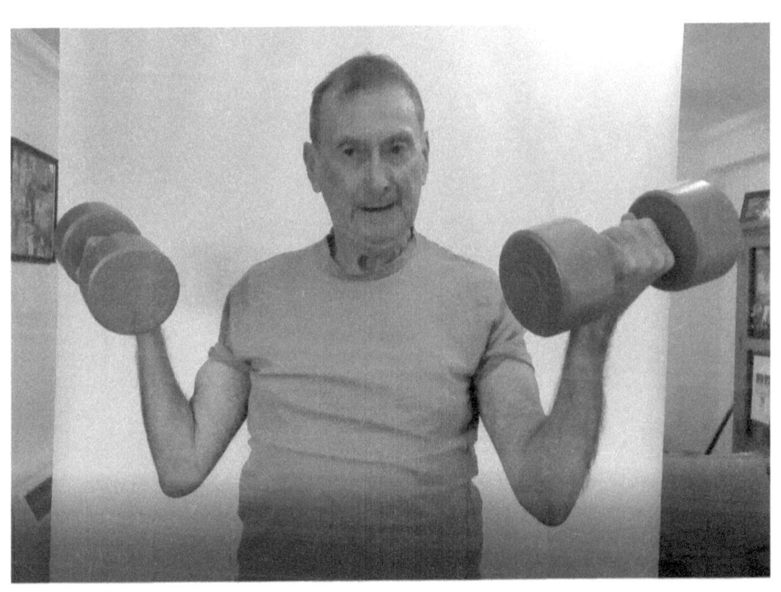

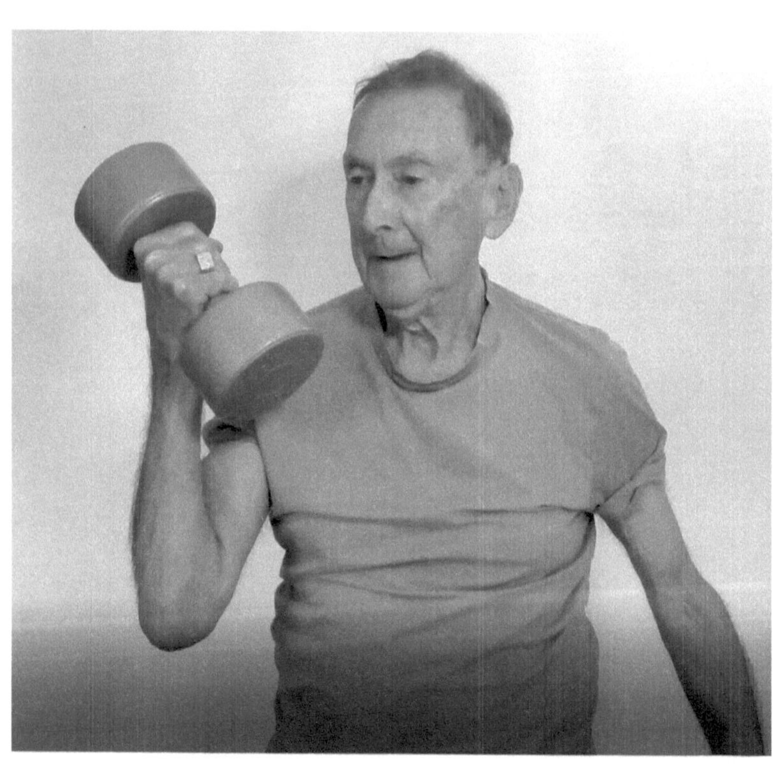

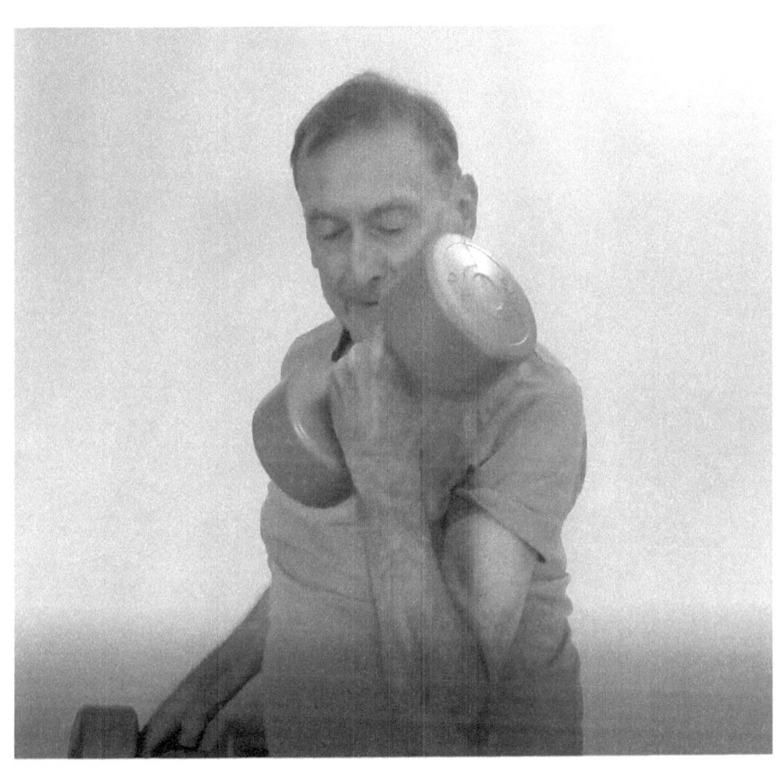

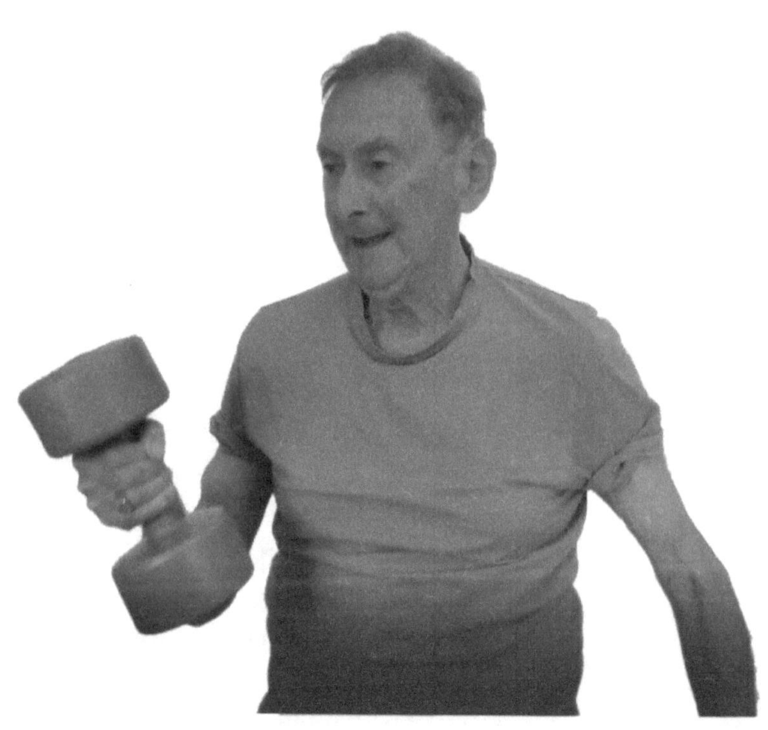

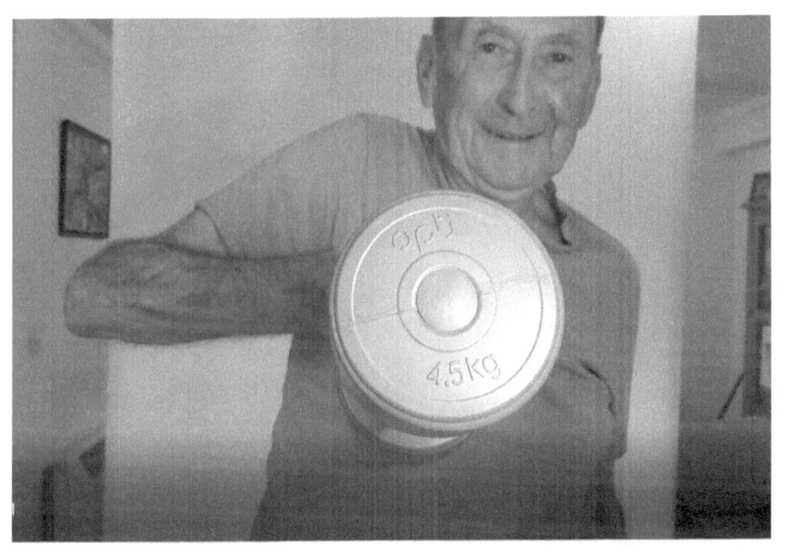
opti
4.5kg

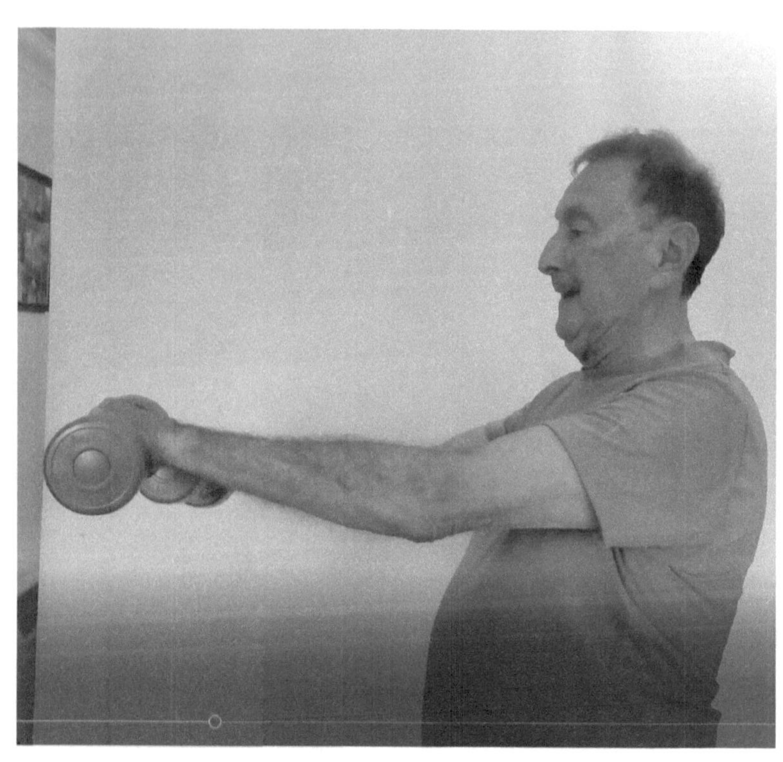

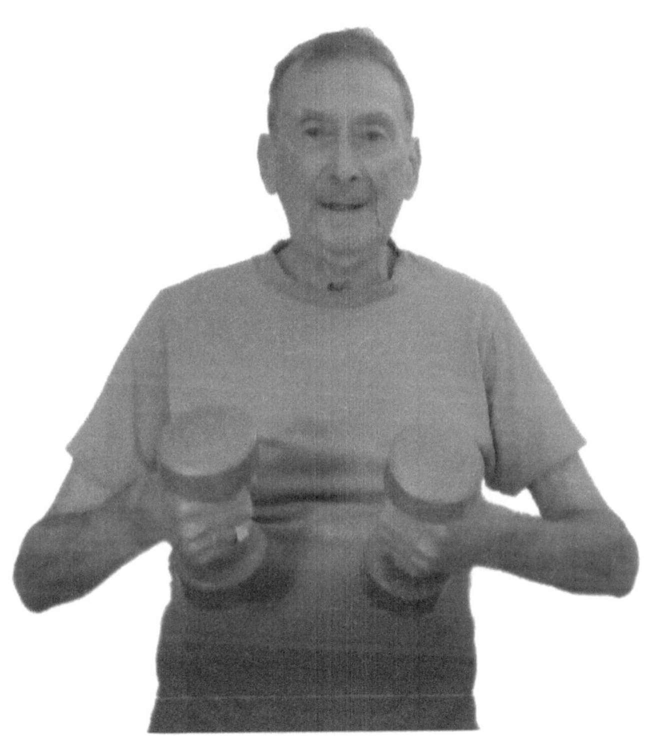

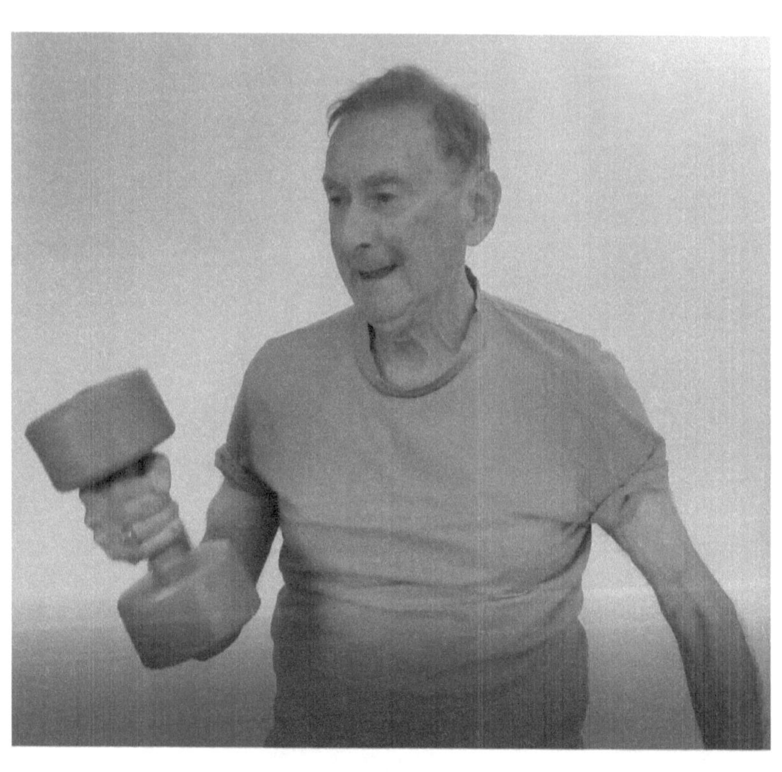

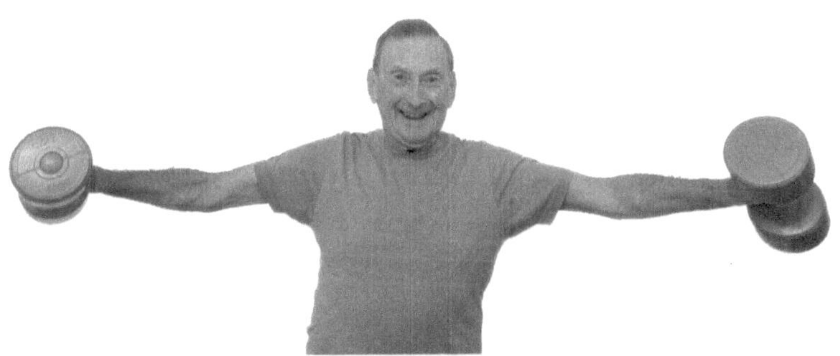

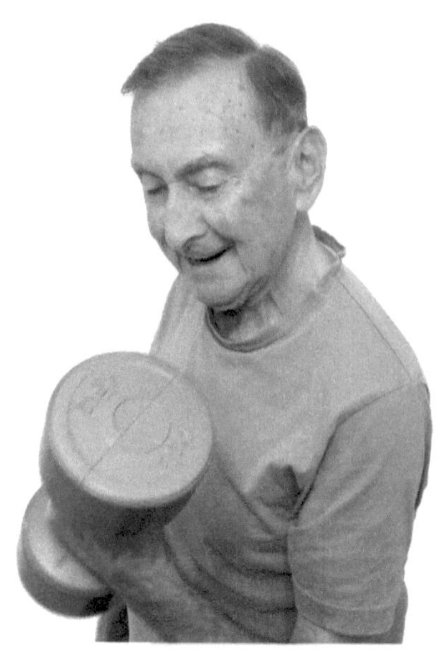

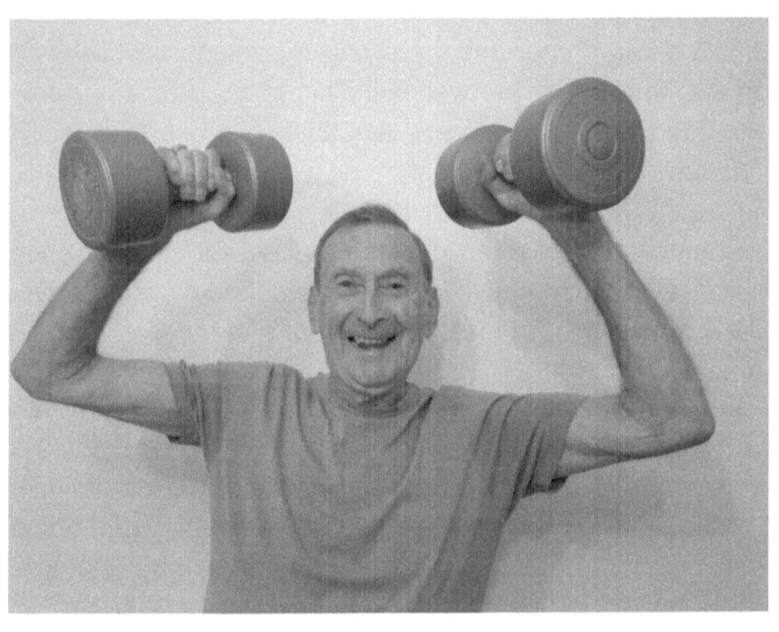

All my organs are functioning well, even the genitalia. I have no arthritis or rheumatism, and no osteoporosis (bone thinness) which is often found in people of my age. I would suggest you keep a set of comfortable clothing, such as a track suit, specifically for exercising, to get you into the right mind-set. It sounds irrelevant but it isn't because we don't always feel like exercising, and putting on a particular outfit can put you into the right mood for it.

I vary the exercises I do each day with the weights, in order to use different muscles. I also use a yoga mat, while lying on the floor, to lift the weights. This is good for the back, shoulders and legs. There are lots of books that teach you how to use free weights, as well as lessons taught on YouTube. Build up an exercise routine of your own. Remember to give yourself a few minutes rest between each exercise, in order to give your heart a chance to slow down. Don't exercise for at least one hour after a meal.

I suggest the workout frequency should be once a week up to age 60, Twice a week from 60 to 70. Three times a week from 70 to 80, and every day from 80+. Sometimes I exercise twice a day, especially if I feel stiff after sitting watching TV in the evening. I find a short workout before I go to bed, for about 20 minutes, helps me sleep better. Of course there are other workouts you can do at bedtime that are just as good if you have a partner, but I won't go into that. Do as much walking as you can, every day if possible. A good rule is to get breathless at least three times a week, no matter how old you are, or irrespective of how you do it. This will strengthen your heart. I gave my lady friend a pair of the 1 kilo weights that I don't use anymore. She has been exercising with them for about a month, and she says she's feeling a whole lot better and stronger already.

MORTALITY

It is said that a woman has an eight year built-in physical advantage over a man as far as mortality is concerned. It is certainly true that men have something like a 20 to 30 per cent higher mortality rate than women in almost every country in the world. However, some men do live to extreme ages. The question is why, and how can more men live longer? Also, just surviving is not particularly desirable, it's only worthwhile if one is physically and mentally active. For example, I know of a man who was a major in the Indian army during the First World War who lived until he was 117 years old. He had a farm at the base of the Himalayas, which he walked around every day, and oversaw the work. Until one day, he decided it was enough, said goodbye to everybody, went to sleep and died.

He had lived a purposeful, active life, in a clean environment, eating only organically grown food. Of course, they were perfect conditions, and we can't expect to emulate that, but a lot can be done, and it can be effective. Even if we don't live to 117, wouldn't it be better to have an active life right up to the end, whenever that is, rather than spending your last days or possibly years, sitting in an armchair in a care home relying on other people for all your needs, and 'waiting for God'?

SLEEP

Sleeping well is very important, it regenerates the batteries. Many older people have problems with sleeping. A lot of them take sleeping tablets. I sometimes have problems sleeping, particularly when I've had a short nap in the afternoon, but I never need to take sleeping pills. After doing some logical thinking on this matter, I came up with a successful method of not only getting to sleep, but getting a good sound sleep for at least 6 hours. First I came to the realisation that the best sleep people have is after they've had a long hard physically or mentally taxing day and are exhausted. Now older people rarely get those sort of days. They're sitting down more and relaxing, often watching TV at night, and then going directly to bed, or having a drink of tea or coffee. These are the worst drinks to have at night as they both contain caffeine which is a stimulant. Even decaf contains small amounts of caffeine. After watching TV at night, I get up and, if I want a hot drink, it will just be boiled water. You can put lemon in boiled water which helps your immune system. Then I do some exercises, sometimes I even play music and do some dancing, I often do push ups to make me feel tired. I try to be in bed by 10.30. I also get up early at the same time every day including weekends, even if I go to bed later. Don't lay in bed and go to sleep again.

I start doing exercises and some weight training for about 20 minutes. This has a number of benefits. It gets the blood circulating around the body. It flexes the muscles, and not only makes you physically tired, but helps to clear the mind, which is very important when you're trying to go to sleep. If you are still lying awake after half-an-hour, get yourself in a comfortable position. Breathe in slowly as you count to 20 or until your lungs are reasonably full, then hold it there, and start counting again from one. When you can no longer hold your breath, release it, remembering how many you have counted. Try to visualise the numbers you are counting. Now exhale as much as you possibly can, and hold it for 10 seconds, then repeat, (breathe in for a count of 20 etc.) Do this four times. On the last exhale just relax everything, and you will be asleep in about 15 minutes or less, and wake up in the morning feeling really refreshed.

SKIN

In this context it's good to be vain. Always remember that as you get older, your body stops producing the oils that feed the skin. It's these oils that keep us smooth and flexible. They also protect the skin from the elements, and give it colour. So you have to replace it with something else. I use various products. In the summer I put on sunscreen every day, on my face and arms. I also use bio-oil and E45 to get rid of the marks on my face. I use coconut cream on the rest of my body. One shouldn't forget the feet which are so important to keep you mobile. Cream the feet and the legs regularly with a recommended cream of some sort. They are the key to keeping you active. I shave every other day, to give my skin a bit of a rest.

STRESS

There are other factors to consider in order to have a happy and healthy life in old age. A good mental attitude is essential. Older people tend to attach too much importance to minor problems, and don't get their priorities right. Keep as organised as possible, if you're having trouble get help. There are organisations such as 'Age Concern' that can be very helpful. Try and develop habits for keeping objects like keys and glasses in the same places as older people's memories are notoriously bad. I have a small plastic box with an alphabetical filing system where I keep my most important information, which I find very useful, and can be bought quite cheaply. You shouldn't let money problems take too much importance in your mind. One doesn't have to be wealthy to enjoy old age, but it is important to have sufficient funds for your needs to avoid major stress. In fact having too much money can be equally harmful. Wealthy people tend to overindulge themselves, and their lives can also be complicated with responsibilities.

SOCIALISING

Loneliness is one of the worst problems, it causes depression which is the biggest enemy of longevity. I have known of millionaires in mansions and living on their own most of the time, who are lonely and miserable.

Human beings are gregarious creatures by nature. We are not meant to be alone. We originally lived together in tribes. These days too many people live a lonely existence, which can cause depression, and also lead to dementia. Socialising, conversation, and laughter is important. Try to join an organisation or social club where you can chat to people and have a joke, or even a disagreement with them. I joined a bowling green club, which allowed me to socialise and keep fit, and was also something my wife and I could do together. If you are not interested in doing any sort of sport, join some sort of support club or organisation. Maybe joining a fan club, or belonging to a political party might interest you. Voluntary work can be very rewarding too. Whatever you do, it is essential to mix with others to stimulate the brain, and help to improve memory, and to avoid loneliness.Try and watch more comedy shows on TV because laughter is very good for you too.

MUSIC

Music has helped me a lot in my life. It can create a cheerful atmosphere when I am feeling depressed, or put me in any mood I choose. It stimulates my brain like nothing else. I can remember music and lyrics that I haven't heard in over seventy years. I am always playing my CDs of which I have quite a large collection from jazz to opera, but my favourites are the swing compositions from the 1930s to the 1970s. I play tracks almost every morning, and often play some jazz to dance to on my own in the evenings, which helps to keep me flexible. I also like to sing in the shower which strengthens the lungs, and the vocal cords. I am learning to play guitar which is fun and good for brain and hand co-ordination. I understand there are MP3s and downloadable music but I'm not into technology like some of you young'uns of 60.

MY LIFE AT 85

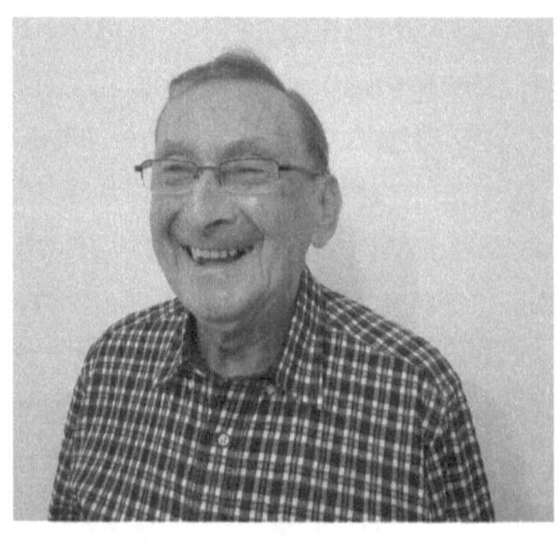

I live on my own in an apartment of a managed retirement block for the over fifty-fives. I look after myself and do all my own shopping, cleaning, and cooking. I am a widower, but I have a lady friend who is a widow and lives in the same block as me. I do my regular daily workouts, and we go walking nearly every day together. I am still driving, and we go somewhere interesting most weeks. We often drive to the coast to visit various seaside towns. We enjoy walking in the country. We both like ballroom dancing and jiving, and we enjoy each other's company. I have played bowls on a bowling green since I was 65 and I still play, weather permitting, and this has kept me flexible and fit as well. My late wife and I have made many friends through bowling over the years in England and in Spain where we used to live. Our married son, with his wife and son lives 15 minutes' drive from me, and we usually meet up every Sunday to go walking, or go on an excursion of some sort. I can still walk miles. I can still swim well. I play bowls, I play snooker, I sing at karaoke, I play guitar, and am still enjoying life. I wouldn't have experienced any of this without my physical fitness. So look after yourself, and enjoy the rest of your life. As my late sister-in-law used to say, "Live long and shit strong !"

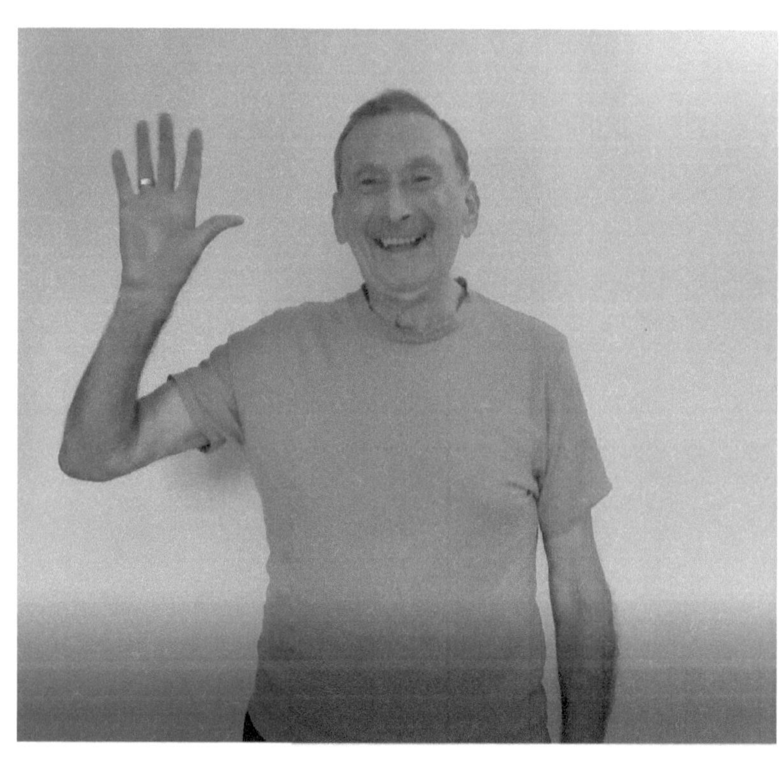

*NOT THE END -
THE BEGINNING*